I0435799

Joy of Living

Mind Body and Soul Wellness Series – Vol 1

Dr. Alka Khurana

Dr. Alka Khurana

To

Our Creator

The One

To Whom We Owe

Everything

Dr. Alka Khurana

My biggest gratitude to God for giving me this opportunity to share my insight on discovering His presence as Joy and Peace within all of us, and my heartiest thanks to my family, friends, loved ones, and well-wishers for their continued support and motivation!

- Alka Khurana

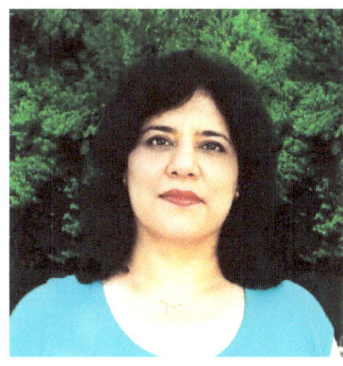

Dr. Alka Khurana is a certified holistic health practitioner and registered medical practitioner in alternative medicine. She teaches techniques to awaken and use the self-healing energy for physical, mental and emotional well-being. She has been practicing Yoga and Meditation for more than 20 years and, during this time she has learnt and practiced many techniques for self-awakening, healing and meditation with various teachers. Based on her extensive experience in healing and meditation, she has designed "Divine Energy Yoga" classes for stress reduction, energy rejuvenation and heightened awareness. Daily practice of these techniques leads one on the path of self-healing and self-realization. She helps people achieve mind, body and soul wellness through the practice of these healing techniques.

She is a Reiki Master Teacher and SUJOK Therapist. She teaches these healing modalities to empower people with tools and techniques to heal themselves at all levels. All these techniques can be used in conjunction with conventional medical treatment, and they complement the conventional medicine by accelerating the healing process. She also provides distant healing to people, if needed, and always encourages everyone to participate in their well-being by learning and practicing the self-healing techniques. She is a wellness coach and provides counseling in good nutrition, stress management, emotional health and dealing with challenging situations.

She also creates spiritual and psychedelic art that brings peace and harmony. She has a Bachelor's degree in Information Technology and Diploma in Visual Arts. She considers Art as one of the ways to connect with the divine energy and higher consciousness. Art is meditation for her and the spiritual knowledge has always guided her in her endeavor. She specializes in Spiritual Art, Yantras, Energy Patterns and several other forms of Healing Arts. She always wishes her art to glow with the aura of liveliness & abundance, and bring joy, peace and healing to everyone. More information about her work in healing and art is available on her websites:

http://DivineEnergyYoga.com, http://SacredArtOnline.com

Preface

Joy is a virtue possessed by all of us. It is not something to be found in the outside world. We have the capacity to feel joyous in an instant, because it always lies within all of us and can be accessed any moment we wish so. The more we know our self and feel connected to our self, the more we experience the joy of living. If we feel happy and joyous, we ignore small undesirable conditions of our life and focus more on the positive things, and the situation gets reversed, if we are feeling sad or upset. So, the state of our being influences our outlook towards our life conditions. One may feel rich and abundant even in the absence of good money, if the heart is filled with Joy and Love. We must always be grateful for whatever life brings to us, and have faith in our self. We can bring happiness to others only if we feel happy and fulfilled in our life. If we celebrate each moment of our life and spread love and happiness in the Universe, the same comes back to us. If we live with positive state of mind we attract more abundance in our life. Our body always follows our mind, and we become healthy at physical level also. Life becomes enjoyable and peaceful.

We are all unique creations of God, constantly learning and growing to express the essence of Divine within all of us. This book is all about discovering the Pure Love and Joy within us, so that we feel more fulfilled in our life and contribute towards the growth of our self as well as others around us. I wish all the readers to experience the Joy of living throughout their journey of life.

May God bless all of us with the vision to be able to see His light in our self and everybody else!

Dr. Alka Khurana

Table of Contents

Dr. Alka Khurana

1: Everyday Spirituality

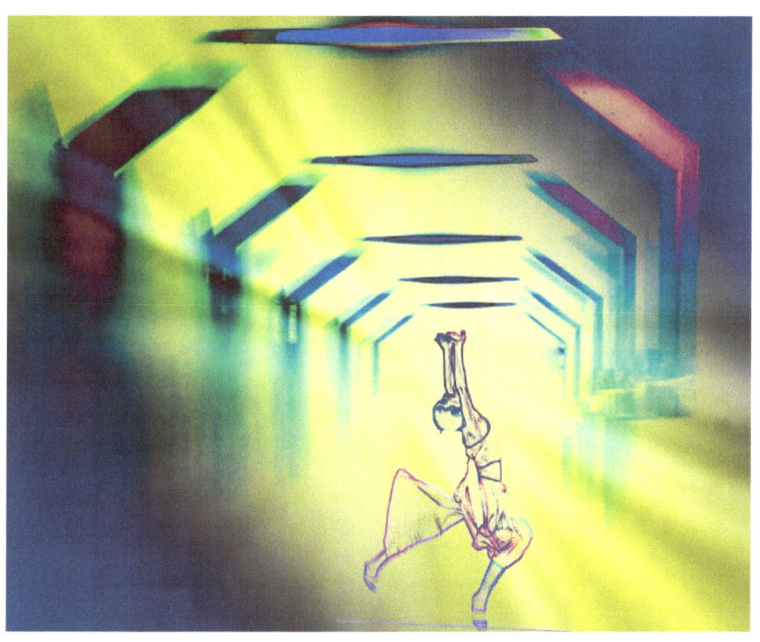

http://sacredartonline.com

"Just as treasures are uncovered from the earth, so virtue appears from good deeds, and wisdom appears from a pure and peaceful mind. To walk safely through the maze of human life, one needs the light of wisdom and the guidance of virtue."

-Buddha

Spirituality is considered as a journey to our own inner self. The essence of spirituality is the search to know our real self and to discover the true nature of our consciousness. It emphasizes on development of positive virtues like unconditional love, compassion, tolerance, forgiveness, contentment, harmony, and empathy towards others. Spirituality helps us to develop inner peace and discover the essence of our own being. It is possible to look at spirituality another way, as something free of institutional structures and hierarchies. It is centered on the deepest values and meanings by which we live, regardless of our faith and religion.

Every day we can take small steps on this path to discover more about our inner realities. We can explore new ways to attain inner peace, joy and fulfillment. Meditation practice helps us to relax our body and calm our mind, to be able to achieve deep states of inner peace. When we follow the guidance of our inner self, change becomes a natural part of our being and we change gracefully, step by step. Without change, there can be no growth, and self-improvement should be our life long mission. Every living thing either grows or dies, that's the law of nature. So, we have to make a continuous effort to know our Self better, and bring about change in order to realize our full potential.

Each one of us is gifted with special talents and unique characteristics. We were all born as instruments of God, and we have to use our special talents for the growth of others. God made each one of us to serve a special purpose contributing to the growth and evolution of humanity. We are a unique creation of God, and we must spread the fragrance of our being in the world around us. Earth is a spiritual battleground, and every day we have to make choices. We must be strong enough to be able to choose light when darkness is overwhelming. Our destiny is shaped by the decisions we make and we are completely responsible for the creation of our life's circumstances.

Spiritual blessings come to us in the form of loyal friends, a loving family, special talents, psychic abilities, healing powers, good health, inner strength, inventions and discoveries for the service of mankind etc. We should be grateful to God for all the blessings and bravely make the right choices in our daily life. Spirituality is not about gaining paper knowledge, rather it's a way of leading our life wisely every single day. It's about realizing the Divinity within our self and connecting with all fellow beings at the same level. Each moment of our life should be filled with joy and happiness, regardless of the external circumstances. A Spiritual person is the one who is always joyous and grateful to the Almighty for His blessings.

Dr. Alka Khurana

2: Mind over Body

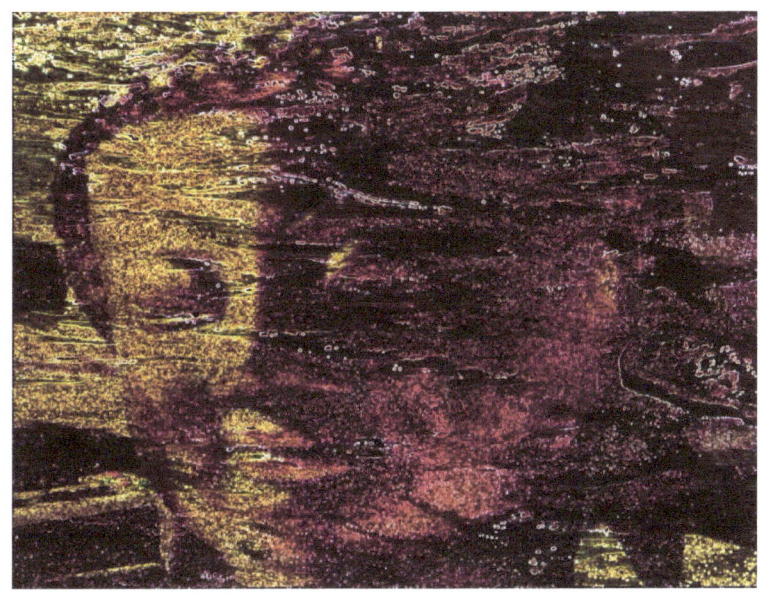

http://sacredartonline.com

"We are shaped by our thoughts; we become what we think. When the mind is pure, joy follows like a shadow that never leaves."

-Buddha

Our body always follows our mind and in order to achieve good health we have to take care of our body as well as our mind. Whenever, we think about good health, we think about good nutrition and regular exercise. These are definitely required to achieve good health, but in addition we need to focus on releasing negative emotions, and experiencing positive states of mind regularly. Our mind is much more powerful in influencing the internal functioning of our body. Based on our mental state, various chemicals are secreted in our body that structure the physical condition of our body. So, we constantly shape our physical well-being based on the thoughts and emotions we feel or imagine on a regular basis.

There is a natural intelligence built in our body to maintain our good health. Our body is constantly breaking the old cells and making the new ones without any conscious instructions being fed to do so. Given a chance, our body has the complete ability to recover itself from any illness. All the healing mechanism is naturally built into our system for proper functioning of our body, but sometimes, due to constant dwelling in undesirable states of mind, we disrupt our well-being and develop some kind of disease/illness. Whenever, we are experiencing any negative state of mind like fear, jealousy, anger, anxiety etc., our body automatically secretes some chemicals that have adverse effects on our internal organs. If we regularly experience or imagine such negative states, lot of toxins get collected in our internal system that need to be cleansed to achieve good health. The tendency to disease and physical disharmony also increases in such situations. However, if we constantly dwell in positive mental states, our body automatically secretes the chemicals that help in building healthy new cells.

Meditation and Energy Healing techniques help in fostering positive states of mind and promote healing. These should be made part of our lifestyle along with good nutrition and physical exercise. We have to cleanse our mental-emotional body daily in the same manner as we cleanse our physical body. This helps in releasing of stored thoughts and emotions of anger, resentment, insult, jealousy etc. and we experience a state of pure love and joy. All the negative states are like clouds, which could be dispelled by the power of wisdom, and then we can see the light of pure love shining within all of us. Our personality can be refined through the exercise of positive mental action in the body, and this helps in increase in our energy and joy of living. The tendency to disease and disharmony decreases and we become more and more perfect beings through which the limitless possibilities of the Divine within may be expressed.

Dr. Alka Khurana

3: Power of Prayers

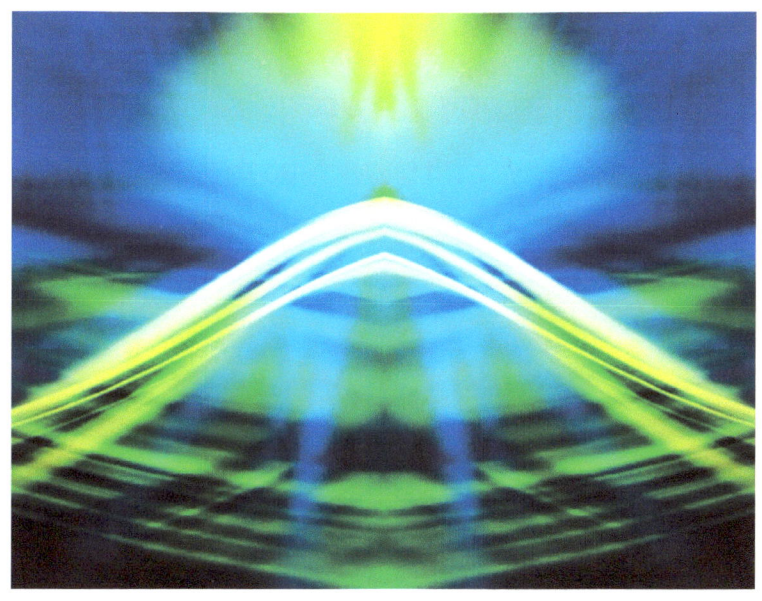

http://sacredartonline.com

"Sometimes, all it takes is just one prayer to change everything."

One of the most important aspect of spirituality is prayer. Prayers help us put our spirituality in action and build inner strength. Words saturated with sincerity, faith conviction carry very high vibrations and they have the power to shatter rocks of difficulty and create the desired change. We must pray to God with the right attitude as His beloved children and always believe that all our prayers are being answered. Prayer has to be sincere directly from the heart and with love to God. The sincerity and faith in our prayer is what gives it the power. The answering of our prayers is in the form of inner strength, guidance, positive thinking and healing energy which help us deal with the challenges of life. Each prayer has a vibration/energy, and when we make positive affirmations, we create positive energy for our self and the people around us. We remain calm even during tough times and move forward with positive attitude.

God gave us the free "will" to lead our life the way we wish. We have to ask for His guidance and protection, otherwise we shall not receive it. We must make positive affirmations to draw more healing power from the source of all creation. We can pray anytime and anywhere as long as we do so with full concentration and sincerity. Our mind should be focused and not wandering elsewhere. We must feel totally relaxed and pray slowly with complete understanding of what we are asking for. It is more beneficial to pray just after rising in the morning and just before going to sleep at night. Our subconscious mind is more awake at this time, and repeated positive affirmations slowly get lodged into it and influence our thoughts and actions. We automatically get directed to perform the right actions needed to manifest our prayers. The stronger the intent, the faster is the manifestation. We can repeat a prayer/affirmation for as many times as desired, but we must repeat it at least three times.

Here is a simple prayer that can be repeated three or more times every morning and evening or whenever possible during the day.

"May we be safe and protected.

**May we be peaceful and
happy.
May we be healthy and strong.
May we always experience
well-being.
Thank You, God Almighty."**

Dr. Alka Khurana

4: Energy Healing

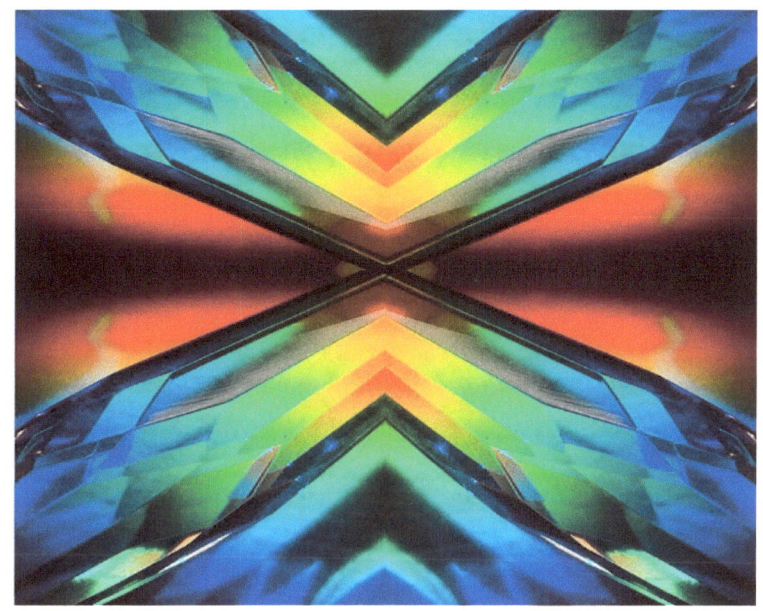

http://sacredartonline.com

"May we always feel the Joy of living!"

The word "heal" comes from the same root-meaning "whole, complete" and "holy". Our body is strongly connected with our internal health maintaining intelligence, which constantly keeps repairing and healing the body. It originates in a space within our innermost being and is the common basis of all healing. We think that we are healed by various systems of medicine and therapy, whether modern or traditional, but, the truth is that the real healer lies within us only. All these healing systems just create the environment where the internal healer gets the best possible conditions to do the healing work. No doctor ever caused a cut on the skin to repair. The inner healing intelligence directed the clotting of blood, the development of scar tissue and new skin. However, the physician may act as a facilitator and by his care some complications in the healing process may be avoided.

Our body tries very hard to put everything back in rightful place and we have to understand that the disease is not a random event, but a distinct message that we deviated from the path of connecting with our true self. Whenever, we are not in compliance with our environment, or we don't feel at ease with some external conditions, we start putting stress on our internal system. Slowly we start developing some illness, which is simply our body's natural effort to get rid of some unwanted internally felt dis-ease. So, whenever we feel physically unwell, there is some obstruction in the internal energy flow of our body. These obstructions are created when some biochemical products start accumulating in the body   at a specific area. This happens because every emotion generates biochemical energy in the body, and these end-products of emotions affect the internal functioning of the body.

The wisdom of Vedas identifies pain as an obstruction to the free flow of joy/energy within and source of all disease is indigestion. This indigestion is physical as well as mental and emotional. So, whenever, there is any stuck emotional input in our mental-emotional body, it manifests itself as pain in our physical body. So, we have to process (digest or eliminate) all such stored emotions to attain the state of good health and wellness. Without releasing such stored energies and just taking medication for physical relief, may result in better physical health for short time only, since the problem still exists in the emotional body. For example, if there is an emotional problem within, it manifests itself as a coronary heart disease. Now, when we perform surgery, it repairs the physical body and creates more suitable conditions for us to understand the underlying emotional distress and deal with the root cause of the illness.

We have to understand how emotional energy works and how Energy Healing deals with it. Ancient healers also explored these areas and shared their findings based on their observations. Dr. Mikao Usui in Japan rediscovered the art of energy healing which is known as Reiki meaning Universal Life-force Energy. Through the regular practice of Energy Healing, we slowly dissolve the blockages present in our mental-emotional body, which results in manifestation of peace and harmony in the whole being.

5: Let us Celebrate Life!

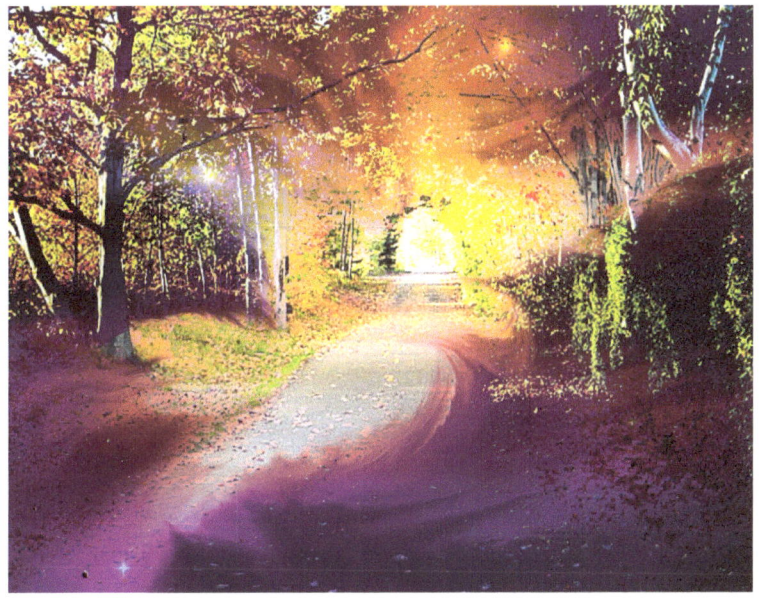

http://sacredartonline.com

"You can search throughout the entire universe for someone who is more deserving of your love and affection than you are yourself, and that person is not to be found anywhere. You yourself, as much as anybody in the entire universe deserve your love and affection."

-Buddha

Modern society has changed the meaning of living for many people. Every day, we are running around to fulfill our immediate needs or some goals of life. Everyone seems to be rushing through life and short on time. We don't find it important to pause and think *"Are we really Living or just Existing?"* Because of society's pressures and some forced upon needs, we have somehow forgotten to lead a meaningful life experiencing every little moment in our journey through life.

There is a common saying that *we only live once*, but to be able to feel *Alive* we have to experience every moment of our life every single day. Each moment of our life is very precious, so instead of dwelling in the past or being anxious about our future, we should learn to enjoy in the present only. Every present moment is quickly going to move into the past, and we have to be always present *here and now* to be able to experience each moment of our life.

"It is better to travel well than to arrive."
-Buddha

We constantly keep thinking that we will be happy when we get so and so, but the truth is that we can get happiness only by feeling happy in the present moment. *"Like attracts like"* is the Universal Law of nature. Only our positive vibrations sent out to the Universe can bring back the same to us. Sometimes, when our goals are not being met or we have to bear some financial or personal loss, we lose hope in our future and start feeling anxious or depressed. Such feelings either keep dragging us into our past or keep us constantly worry about our future. We perceive such situations as difficult and challenging, but actually this is God's way of giving us the opportunity to grow and learn. Life is a *Learning School*, and we have to constantly keep learning from our experiences throughout our life. We must have full faith in His decisions and lead our life with love and wisdom.

Life is a precious gift from God Almighty. When we rush through it, we miss on the *Joy of Living*. Let's celebrate every moment of our life irrespective of our surrounding environment or conditions. Let's be present in each moment and enjoy every step of our journey without thinking about the destination.

Dr. Alka Khurana

6: Daily Practice to attract Abundance

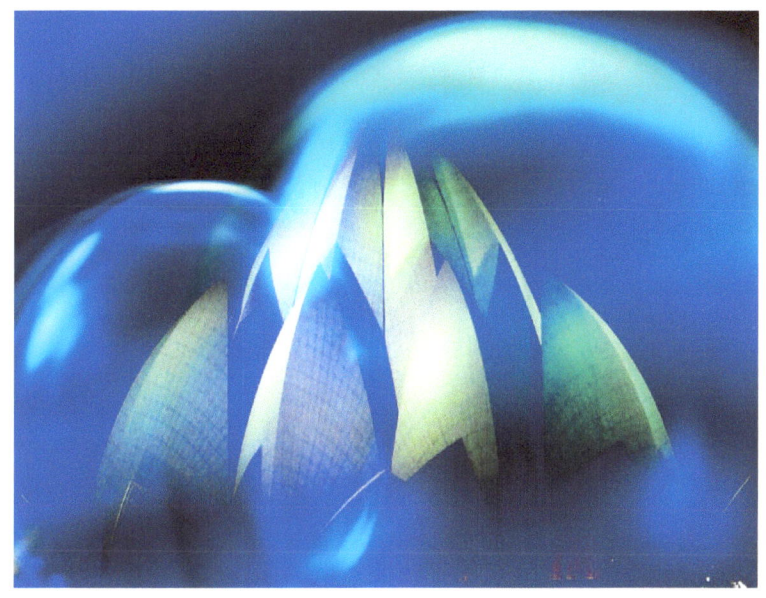

http://sacredartonline.com

"Let us be Alive in every moment of our life"

Here is a 5 minute exercise which can be practiced every night before going to sleep. It will bring us in a positive state of mind, and while we are sleeping our subconscious mind will automatically work to bring more abundance in our life.

It is a two-step exercise:

Step 1: We must think about any three good things that happened today. It can be anything mundane or most exalted, but it should seem to bring more abundance and happiness in our life. It can be as simple a fact like "I enjoyed the evening walk today" or something else like "I was announced the #1 bestseller author." We can either write down such three good things from the day or we may contemplate them mentally.

Step 2: Next is the very important part of this exercise where we must reflect on "why" each good thing happened. We have to find the reason for each event and feel the gratitude towards the people or conditions involved. For example, I enjoyed the walk because God gave me the strength to go out, or maybe because two strangers greeted me with a smile, or maybe because the weather was so pleasant, or whatever else that made your walk enjoyable. It can be any reason that makes sense to us. Let's now extend our love and gratitude to God or other people involved in bringing those happy moments in our life today. Let's feel that love and peace completely with a big smile on our face and close the day with this small prayer to God.

"Oh God, protect us from all negativity,
Fill our heart with eternal love and peace,
Keep us healthy and always guide us with your light.
Thank you God!"

7: How to handle life's challenges

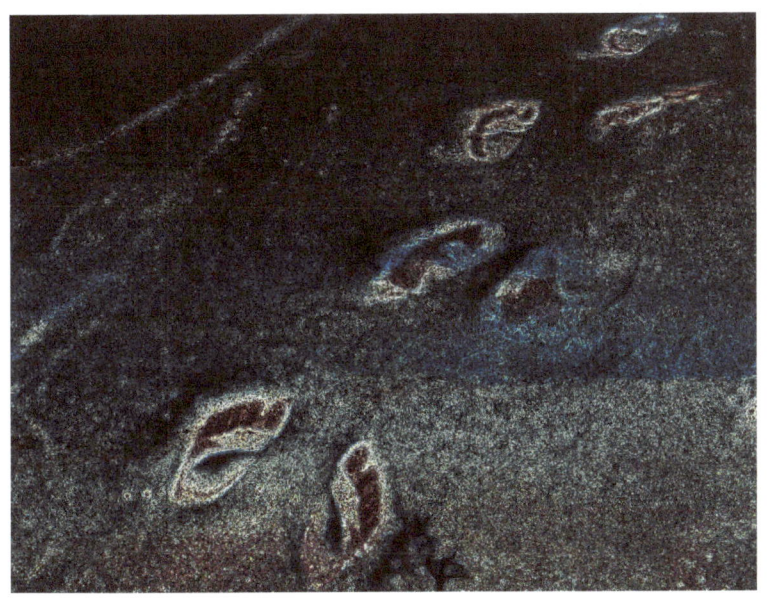

http://sacredartonline.com

"Let's know and embrace our true self"

Life is a journey which we can complete either by complaining about the challenges, or by gracefully accepting them as an opportunity to learn and grow. We are constantly conditioned to avoid pain and work towards getting more happiness in life. Whenever, we perceive us going through difficult time, we get angry/sad and keep waiting for that time to end. However, life passes in moments and we must completely live every moment regardless of the feeling that it brings. Happiness or sorrow, both is transient states and the only thing that's permanent in life is "change". Good or bad times are just the perceptions of our mind. Here is a great Mantra to be remembered:

"This too will pass."

We should always remember this mantra, and not get attached to any event of our life. If we always remember this mantra, nothing can make us suffer in our life and we can always be satisfied with whatever life brings to us. If we follow this mantra, we shall never get overwhelmed in any situation and lead our life with peace and gratitude.

Our life is directed by the inner desires stored in our subconscious mind i.e. our "feeling mind". Here so many of our desires are deeply rooted, which drive us towards the various experiences of our life. Each event of our life is extremely important for our growth and development. Present moment is the only time that's real and to be lived completely. Therefore, we should calmly lead our life, gracefully accepting each experience as a gift from God and, without getting attached to any experience; we should keep reminding our self that "This too will pass".

8: Good or Bad

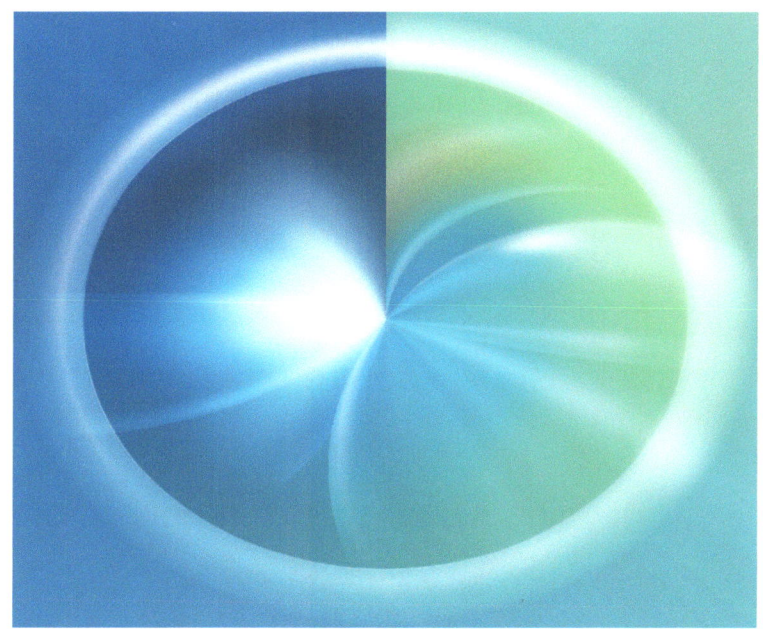

http://sacredartonline.com

"Oh Lord! May we always see Your light shining in all Your creations."

Good and bad is one like two sides
of the same coin. Every day we label
people and situations as good or bad,
based on our feelings associated with
them. Something that brings us
happiness is labeled as good, and the
reverse is true for bad. But, in reality
there is no absolute good or bad, rather,
it's all relative and depends on the way
our mind associates the feelings of good
or bad to any event in our life.

Every person is a unique
combination of various traits, which
serve him to evolve and learn in this life
time. For example, if someone has to
learn to have more patience, he'll be put
into difficult situations from time to time
until he learns the lesson and develops
the habit of perseverance and tolerance.

Now, during those learning times he may label such situations as bad, even though they are helping him to become a stronger person. So, we look at events as good or bad based on the pain or pleasure we derive from them. And if we think about people, there is no classification as good or bad, as we are all the same. However, each one of us behaves differently (so called good or bad) in different situations based on our conditioning and mental convictions. We are all unique pieces of the one big jigsaw puzzle called the Universe. Each one of us has unique features and all of us are equally important to complete this Universe. All of us have same Divinity and pure love within us. Our inner Self has all the wisdom and is always awake; we just have to listen to its guidance. We shall be able to see the Divine in others only when are able to see it in our Self. If we love our self completely without any judgments, we shall be able to accept everyone else as a unique person made in the image of God. Then our mind stops judging people as good or bad and we start accepting every individual as a beautiful creation of God; and each event of our life as an important stepping stone towards our growth and development.

9: The Golden Rule for Emotional Health

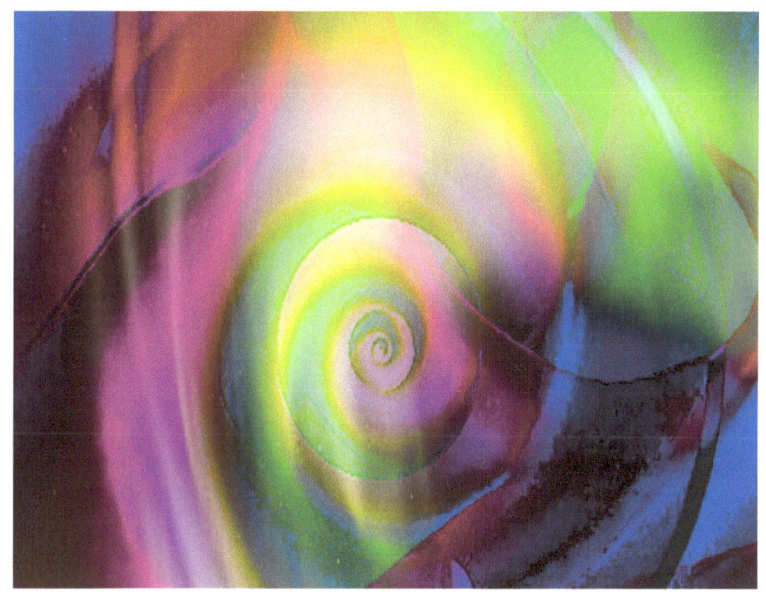

http://sacredartonline.com

"Peace comes from within. Do not seek it without."

- Buddha

Here is a Golden Rule to achieve good emotional health:

"Be a provider of all the emotions you want to experience in life."

Every day we look forward to receive love, respect, happiness etc. from our friends/family/co-workers, and feel disappointed if they are not able to meet our expectations. Now, instead of waiting for their response or permission, we can constantly experience these elated emotions, if we take the initiative to become the provider of these emotions. If we follow this Golden Rule, we can experience positive emotions all the time at our own will. We have to be the change we want to see in others.

"We feel loved, whenever we give love.

We feel respected, whenever we treat others with respect.

We feel inner strength, whenever we help someone.

We feel happy, whenever we appreciate something.

We feel joyous, whenever we thank God for His blessings."

Dr. Alka Khurana

10: Unconditional Love

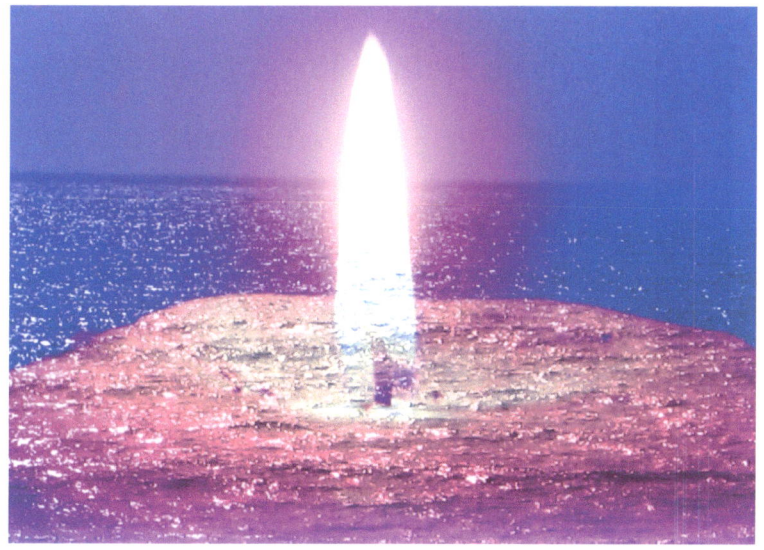

http://sacredartonline.com

"Thousands of candles can be lighted from a single candle, and the life of the candle will not be shortened. Happiness never decreases by being shared."

- Buddha

Love is considered to be the most basic emotion that our consciousness can feel. While experiencing love, we allow the free flow of life force energy in our whole being. We are all searching for true love every moment of our life. Whenever, we get glimpses of such deep love and bonding, we cherish those moments throughout our life. When we share our love with others, we give positive energy to them and also to our self. It is in the sharing and giving of love to others that we receive the same. Express love to the world around you and the world will reflect back to you the power of love.

However, the greatest power known to man is that of unconditional love. We were taught by consistent experience that love was conditional, and we had to buy love from the people around us with our words and behavior. However, unconditional love is a natural expression that does not expect an outcome. It is not determined by the one being loved, but rather by the one choosing to love. This is not the type of love we give to earn favors or love in return; rather, it is giving just for the sake of giving and sharing something that lies within us.

Pure Divine Love is what we all are. It's the unconditional love of God passed on to all His creations. God is always giving love unconditionally to each one of us all the time without judging our actions. Whenever, we receive God's Divine love in our deep prayers, it makes us feel empowered and fills our heart with joy. It's the most powerful and rejuvenating energy that can be felt by our consciousness. Mere thought of love brings smile on our face and we do not always need another person or thing to experience love. It is not to be derived from any outside source, but we all our self are an infinite source of it. Divine Unconditional Love is our essence and it is the eternal wealth that we all inherited from God. We were all made in His image and possess the same qualities. We can perceive our soul/self as a drop from the ocean of omnipresent super-consciousness/God. As the drop has same constituents as the ocean, so we are also same as the God. We have to realize our true nature to be able to experience this powerful force. The easiest way to start experiencing this boundless love energy is to take our attention inwards and start giving unconditional love to our self. We are a unique creation of God, and we should honor God's decision by loving our self without any judgment or conditions. We just have to let it flow freely through us, and the more we share, the more it empowers us.

"Let's realize the presence of Divine Unconditional Love within our heart and share this boundless energy with everyone around us.

Dr. Alka Khurana

11: Meditate to experience Joy

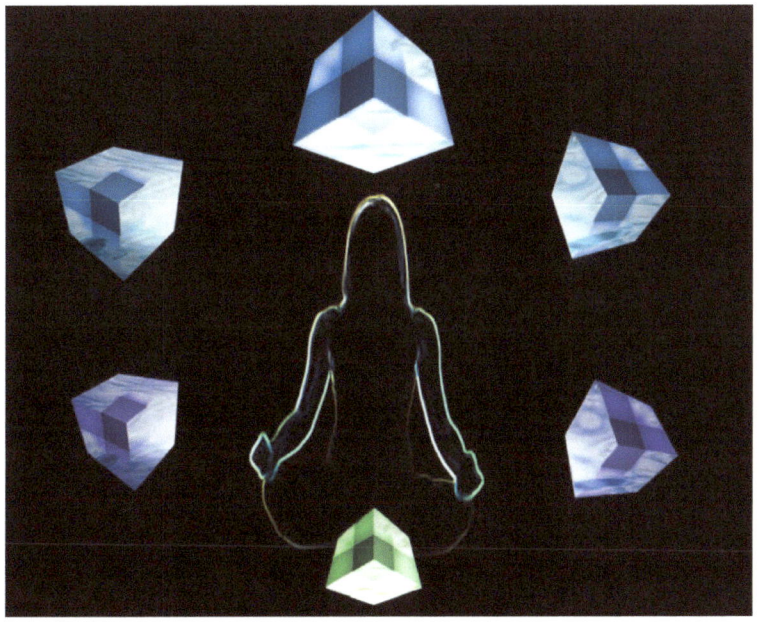

http://sacredartonline.com

"When even one virtue becomes our nature, the mind becomes clean and tranquil. Then there is no need to practice meditation; we will automatically be meditating always."

— Swami Satchidananda

Meditation is a state of intense awareness achieved by stillness of our thoughts. It's a journey to the center of own being, and experiencing our natural state of expanded awareness.
Meditation helps us to relax and allows us to discover truths about our own nature. Meditation is all about being completely in the present moment and letting go of any past or future. We simply have to drop all our thoughts and put aside the mental tendency to constantly worry and plan.

We all possess three states of thinking - conscious thinking during the waking state, subconscious during deep sleep and super-conscious during self-awareness. Meditation is not a passive state of daydreaming or drifting in a sub consciousness state, rather, it brings us in touch with the super-conscious state of intense awareness. When we are able to internalize the energy of our senses during meditation, it awakens a tremendous flow of energy in our whole being. We are able to deeply relax our body and mind, and expand our sense of identity until we realize our unity with all creation.

Meditation has great health benefits and gives us a respite from excessive stress of daily life. As we relax, our blood pressure lowers and our response mechanism slows down. We become more centered and don't react as strongly or negatively to adverse situations. Meditation has been found to strengthen the immune system and enhance the activity of "telomerase" enzyme that protects genetic material during cell division and enhances cellular viability. Consistent meditation practice fosters improvement in emotional well-being and helps release of negative mental states such as fear, anger and worry. We inculcate more positive attitudes and show love and compassion towards every creation of God. We are able to experience the love and joy present within our self, and share it with the world around us; bringing peace and harmony.

12: Technique to release Anger/Anxiety

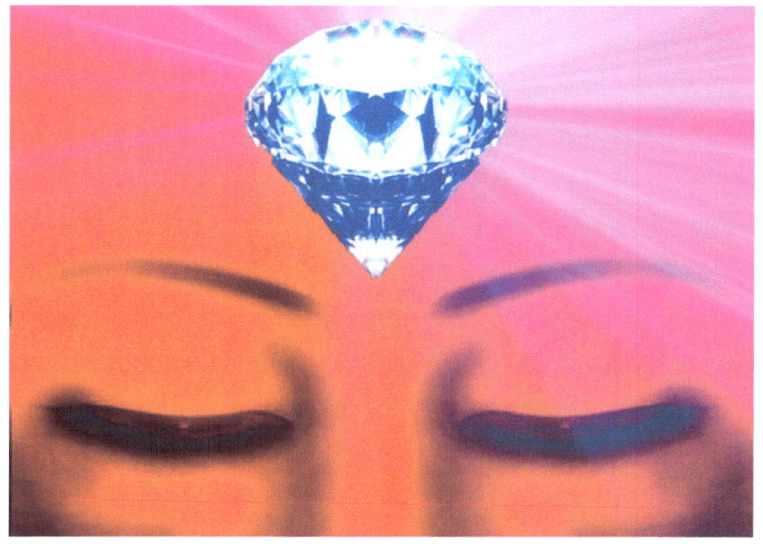

http://sacredartonline.com

"Holding on to anger is like grasping a hot coal with the intent of throwing it at someone else; you are the one who gets burned."

- Buddha

All the emotions like fear, anger, anxiety, jealousy, love, compassion, peace etc. are generated by the same energy center in our body. Same energy is transformed into an empowering or disturbing emotion. We always feel more energetic and resourceful while experiencing/imagining a positive emotion because it increases the flow of prana/life-force energy into our body. On the contrary, in the event of experiencing a negative emotion, we feel weak and depleted because, during that time we block the flow of prana/life-force energy into our body. The nature of our emotion determines the quality of energy flow energy in our body. All emotions are essential for our survival and growth, and it is very natural to experience an array of emotions in our daily life. We should not try to suppress or condemn any natural emotion, rather we should learn the skills to transform any weakening emotion to an empowering one.

We have several energy centers (also called chakras) in our body which act as energy vortices. These centers are located along our spinal column and act as energy transformers in our body to supply the internal organs with life-force energy. The heart center located in the middle of our chest is responsible for all the emotions regarding our relationship with our self and others. A healthy heart chakra allows us to love deeply, feel compassion, and have a deep sense of peace and centeredness.

Whenever the undesirable emotions of fear, anger, hatred or anxiety arise in our heart, we can use the following technique to transform them to empowering states of love, forgiveness, faith and compassion.

This visualization can be performed while sitting comfortably in a straight-back chair or standing or lying down. Close your eyes and let the tips of your index finger and thumb touch. Put your right hand in front of the chest and concentrate on the space in the center of the chest. Take a few slow and deep breaths and visualize a small sphere of while light in that space. Chant the sound "YAM" and imagine that the sphere of light is expanding in size. Keep chanting either mentally or aloud, and let the sphere of light surround your whole body. Let the light get into each cell of your body and be in this sphere of pure white light for as long as you feel comfortable. Feel one with this comforting pure energy and try to bring forward the other person or situation that were triggering the emotions of anger/ hatred/ fear/ anxiety in you. See them also filled with the same pure energy and let them merge with your energy to create a bigger sphere of white light. Accept them as a gift from God and try to listen to God's hidden message through them. Every such situation/person is a true blessing for us to grow as a person and understand the deeper meanings of life.

Give all your fears to this loving light of God and have love, forgiveness and compassion first for yourself and then for others involved. Be thankful to God for this precious gift which helped you to understand and transform your stored emotions within this pure energy sphere. The other person/situation only acts as a trigger to experience the various emotions stored deep within us. Feel the joy and peace within you and see your heart radiating pure white light in all directions. Thank God for sending this purifying white light and let it go back its source. See your heart overflowing with rays of inner peace and joy. Bring both your hands with palms together, in front of your chest and say this phrase three times: "I am love, I am peace", and slowly open your eyes with a smile.

This visualization exercise can also be performed as part of our daily meditation practice to experience love, joy and peace within us.

Dr. Alka Khurana

THANK YOU

www.ingramcontent.com/pod-product-compliance
Lightning Source LLC
Chambersburg PA
CBHW050808290526
45792CB00001B/34